Transitional Year Residency Match Selection Criteria and Programs Requirements.

By

Match A Doc
and
Residency Guide

Table of Contents

Introduction

Transitional Year Residency Match Selection Criteria and Programs Requirements

This book is the must-read book and most single important piece you buy in your battle for residency. This is the Transitional

Year Residency Match Selection Criteria and Programs Requirements book that contains up-to-date information about all the programs in the United States for both AMGs and IMGs. Why this book is essential to match? It has been shown that applying to programs that you don't match their minimum criteria is just waste of money and time. It is very important that you apply to those programs that you meet their requirements and this why we decided to make your life easier by gathering the information you need in one book. The information was gathered from program directors, coordinators, chiefs, faculty and residents. It includes Programs names, Programs codes, States, Addresses, Phones, Faxes, Percentage of IMGs in the programs, Minimum USMLE Step 1 and Step 2 Score Requirements, Attempts on any step, CS requirement at time of application, USCE Requirements, Cut-Off time since graduation, Programs offering couple match and Visas Sponsored or accepted. We have more than 10 years experience in the match field and our book is the proof that will help you to get the highest number of interviews to increase your chances in the match journey.

Alabama

Baptist Medical Center Transitional Year Residency Program

Specialty: Transitional Year
Program name: Baptist Medical Center Program
Program code: 999-01-00-001
NRMP Code: 1903999P0
Program type: Community-based
State: Alabama
Address: Baptist Medical Center Princeton,
817 Princeton Ave SW, Birmingham,
AL 35211
Phone: (205) 783-7663
Fax: (205) 783-7399
Percentage of IMGs in the program: 0%
Minimum USMLE Step 1 Score Requirement:
200
Minimum USMLE Step 2 Score Requirement:
205
Attempts on any step: No limits set
CS required at time of application: No
USCE Requirement: None

Cut-Off time since graduation: 5 years
Program offers couple match: Yes
Visas Sponsored or accepted: J1 visa

Arizona

College of Medicine Mayo Clinic (Arizona) Transitional Year Residency Program

Specialty: Transitional Year
Program name: Mayo Clinic College of Medicine (Arizona) Program
Program code: 999-03-00-226
State: Arizona
Address: Mayo Clinic Hospital, 2W Medical Education,
          5777 E Mayo Blvd, Phoenix, AZ 85259
Phone: (480) 342-2894
Fax: (480) 342-2027
Percentage of IMGs in the program: 0%
Minimum USMLE Step 1 Score Requirement: No limits set
Minimum USMLE Step 2 Score Requirement: No limits set
Attempts on any step: No limits set
CS required at time of application: Yes
including ECFMG certificate

USCE Requirement: None
Cut-Off time since graduation: 5 years
Program offers couple match: Yes
Visas Sponsored or accepted: J1 visa and H1b visa

Tucson Hospitals Medical Education Transitional Year Residency Program

Specialty: Transitional Year
Program name: Tucson Hospitals Medical Education Program
Program code: 999-03-00-006
NRMP Code: 1014999P0
Program type: Community-based university affiliated hospital
State: Arizona
Address: Tucson Hospitals Medical Education Program,

5301 E Grant Rd, Tucson, AZ 85733
Phone: (520) 324-5096
Fax: (520) 324-5231
Percentage of IMGs in the program: 0%
Minimum USMLE Step 1 Score Requirement: 210
Minimum USMLE Step 2 Score Requirement: 210
Attempts on any step: Must pass on first attempt including CS exam

CS required at time of application: No
USCE Requirement: Yes
Cut-Off time since graduation: 2 years
Program offers couple match: Yes
Visas Sponsored or accepted: No visa

California

Kaweah Delta Health Care District (KDHCD) Transitional Year Residency Program

Specialty: Transitional Year
Program name: Kaweah Delta Health Care District (KDHCD) Program
Program code: 999-05-00-244
State: California
Address: Kaweah Delta Health Care District, 400 W Mineral King Ave, Visalia, CA 93291
Phone: (559) 624-5215
Fax: (559) 713-2312
Percentage of IMGs in the program: 0%
Minimum USMLE Step 1 Score Requirement: No limits set
Minimum USMLE Step 2 Score Requirement: No limits set
Attempts on any step: No limits set

CS required at time of application: Yes including ECFMG certificate and PTAL
USCE Requirement: None
Cut-Off time since graduation: 5 years
Program offers couple match: Yes
Visas Sponsored or accepted: J1 visa

Los Angeles County-Harbor-UCLA Medical Center Transitional Year Residency Program

Specialty: Transitional Year
Program name: Los Angeles County-Harbor-UCLA Medical Center Program
Program code: 999-05-00-239
State: California
Address: Los Angeles County-Harbor-UCLA Med Center,
        1000 W Carson St, Torrance, CA 90509
Phone: (310) 222-2903
Fax: (310) 782-8599
Percentage of IMGs in the program: 0%
Minimum USMLE Step 1 Score Requirement: No limits set
Minimum USMLE Step 2 Score Requirement: No limits set
Attempts on any step: No limits set
CS required at time of application: No
USCE Requirement: None

Cut-Off time since graduation: No limits set
Program offers couple match: Yes
Visas Sponsored or accepted: J1 visa

Santa Clara Valley Medical Center Transitional Year Residency Program

Specialty: Transitional Year
Program name: Santa Clara Valley Medical Center Program
Program code: 999-05-00-013
NRMP Code: 1820999P0, 1063999P0
Program type: Community-based university affiliated hospital
State: California
Address: Santa Clara Valley Medical Center, 751 S Bascom Ave, San Jose, CA 95128
Phone: (408) 885-6305
Fax: (408) 885-4046
Percentage of IMGs in the program: 0%
Minimum USMLE Step 1 Score Requirement: No limits set
Minimum USMLE Step 2 Score Requirement: No limits set
Attempts on any step: No limits set
CS required at time of application: Yes including ECFMG certificate and PTAL
USCE Requirement: None

Cut-Off time since graduation: 5 years
Program offers couple match: Yes
Visas Sponsored or accepted: No visa

Scripps Mercy Hospital Transitional Year Residency Program

Specialty: Transitional year
Program name: Scripps Mercy Hospital Program
Program code: 999-05-00-010
NRMP Code: 1048999P0, 1048999P2
Program type: Community-based university affiliated hospital
State: California
Address: Scripps Mercy Hospital,
4077 Fifth Ave, San Diego, CA 92103-2180
Phone: (619) 260-7220
Fax: (619) 260-7305
Percentage of IMGs in the program: 0%
Minimum USMLE Step 1 Score Requirement: No limits set
Minimum USMLE Step 2 Score Requirement: No limits set
Attempts on any step: Must pass on first attempt including CS exam
CS required at time of application: Yes including ECFMG certificate and PTAL
USCE Requirement: None

Cut-Off time since graduation: 5 years
Program offers couple match: Yes
Visas Sponsored or accepted: No visa

Colorado

Colorado Health Foundation Presbyterian-St Luke Medical Center Transitional Year Residency Program

Specialty: Transitional Year
Program name: Colorado Health Foundation Presbyterian-St Luke's Medical Center Program
Program code: 999-07-00-017
NRMP Code: 2065999P0
Program type: Community-based university affiliated hospital
State: Colorado
Address: Colorado Health Foundation-St Luke's Med Center, #520,
           1721 E 19th Ave, Denver, CO 80218
Phone: (303) 869-2093

Percentage of IMGs in the program: 0%

Minimum USMLE Step 1 Score Requirement: 220
Minimum USMLE Step 2 Score Requirement: 220
Attempts on any step: Must pass on first attempt
CS required at time of application: Yes including ECFMG certificate
USCE Requirement: None
Cut-Off time since graduation: No limits set
Program offers couple match: Yes
Visas Sponsored or accepted: None

Connecticut

Yale-New Haven Hospital Transitional Year Residency Program

Specialty: Transitional Year
Program name: Yale-New Haven Hospital Program
Program code: 999-08-00-020
NRMP Code: 1090999P0
Program type: University-based

State: Connecticut
Address: Yale New Haven, Transitional Year Program

        1450 Chapel St, New Haven, CT 06511-4440
Phone: (203) 789-3989
Fax: (203) 789-3222
Percentage of IMGs in the program: 30%
Minimum USMLE Step 1 Score Requirement: No limits set
Minimum USMLE Step 2 Score Requirement: No limits set
Attempts on any step: Must pass on first attempt
CS required at time of application: Yes
USCE Requirement: None
Cut-Off time since graduation: 3 years
Program offers couple match: Yes
Visas Sponsored or accepted: J1 visa

St. Vincent Medical Center Transitional Year Residency Program

Specialty: Transitional Year
Program name: St Vincent's Medical Center Program
Program code: 999-08-00-018
NRMP Code: 1080999P0

Program type: Community-based university affiliated hospital
State: Connecticut
Address: St Vincent's Medical Center, Transitional Year Program,
    2800 Main St, Bridgeport, CT 06606
Phone: 203 576 5578

Percentage of IMGs in the program: 80%
Minimum USMLE Step 1 Score Requirement: 210
Minimum USMLE Step 2 Score Requirement: 210
Attempts on any step: No limits set
CS required at time of application: Yes
USCE Requirement: None
Cut-Off time since graduation: 10 years
Program offers couple match: Yes
Visas Sponsored or accepted: J1 visa and H1b visa

Delaware

Christiana Care Health Services Transitional Year Residency Program

Specialty: Transitional Year

Program name: Christiana Care Health Services Program
Program code: 999-09-00-021
NRMP Code: 1099999P0
Program type: Community-based university affiliated hospital
State: Delaware
Address: Christiana Care Health System, Ammon Education Bldg; Suite 2E70,
          4755 Ogletown-Stanton Rd, Newark, DE 19718
Phone: (302) 733-6338
Fax: (302) 733-6386
Percentage of IMGs in the program: 0%
Minimum USMLE Step 1 Score Requirement: No limits set
Minimum USMLE Step 2 Score Requirement: No limits set
Attempts on any step: No limits set
CS required at time of application: No
USCE Requirement: None
Cut-Off time since graduation: No limits set
Program offers couple match: Yes
Visas Sponsored or accepted: J1 visa and H1b visa

District of Columbia

Georgetown University Hospital Transitional Year Residency Program

Specialty: Transitional Year
Program name: Georgetown University Hospital Program
Program code: 999-51-00-205
NRMP Code: 1801999P0
Program type: Community-based university affiliated hospital
State: District of Columbia
Address: Inova Fairfax Hospital,
            3300 Gallows Rd, Falls Church, VA 22042-3300
Phone: (703) 776-2166
Fax: (703) 776-3020
Percentage of IMGs in the program: 0%
Minimum USMLE Step 1 Score Requirement: 200
Minimum USMLE Step 2 Score Requirement: 205
Attempts on any step: No limits set
CS required at time of application: Yes
USCE Requirement: None
Cut-Off time since graduation: No limits set
Program offers couple match: Yes
Visas Sponsored or accepted: J1 visa

Georgia

The Medical Center Transitional Year Residency Program

Specialty: Transitional Year
Program name: The Medical Center Program
Program code: 999-12-00-229
NRMP Code: 1118999P0
Program type: Community-based
State: Georgia
Address: The Medical Center Inc, Suite 100
        1900 10th Ave, Columbus, GA 31902
Phone: (706) 571-1430
Fax: (706) 571-1604
Percentage of IMGs in the program: 20%
Minimum USMLE Step 1 Score Requirement: No limits set
Minimum USMLE Step 2 Score Requirement: No limits set
Attempts on any step: No limits set
CS required at time of application: Yes
USCE Requirement: None
Cut-Off time since graduation: 5 years
Program offers couple match: Yes
Visas Sponsored or accepted: No

Emory University Transitional Year Residency Program

Specialty: Transitional Year
Program name: Emory University Program
Program code: 999-12-00-026
Program type: University-based
State: Georgia
Address: Grady Memorial Hospital,
49 Jesse Hill Jr Dr SE, Atlanta, GA 30303
Phone: (404) 778-0263
Fax: (404) 778-1601
Percentage of IMGs in the program: 10%
Minimum USMLE Step 1 Score Requirement: 230
Minimum USMLE Step 2 Score Requirement: 230
Attempts on any step: Must pass on first attempt
CS required at time of application: Yes
USCE Requirement: None
Cut-Off time since graduation: 3 years
Program offers couple match: Yes
Visas Sponsored or accepted: J1 visa and H1b visa

Hawaii

University of Hawaii Transitional Year Residency Program

Specialty: Transitional Year
Program name: University of Hawaii Program
Program code: 999-14-00-031
NRMP Code: 3350999P0
Program type: Community-based university affiliated hospital
State: Hawaii
Address: University of Hawaii John A Burns School of Medicine,
          1356 Lusitana St, Honolulu, HI 96813-2427
Phone: (808) 586-7477
Fax: (808) 586-7486
Percentage of IMGs in the program: 0%
Minimum USMLE Step 1 Score Requirement: No limits set
Minimum USMLE Step 2 Score Requirement: No limits set
Attempts on any step: No limits set
CS required at time of application: No
USCE Requirement: Yes
Cut-Off time since graduation: No limits set
Program offers couple match: Yes
Visas Sponsored or accepted: J1 visa

Illinois

St. Francis Hospital of Evanston Transitional Year Residency Program

Specialty: Transitional Year
Program name: Presence St Francis Hospital Program
Program code: 999-16-00-038
NRMP Code: 1168999P0
Program type: Community-based university affiliated hospital
State: Illinois
Address: St Francis Hospital, Department of Medical Education,
 355 Ridge Ave, Evanston, IL 60202
Phone: (847) 316-3111
Fax: (847) 316-3307
Percentage of IMGs in the program: 0%
Minimum USMLE Step 1 Score Requirement: 220
Minimum USMLE Step 2 Score Requirement: 220
Attempts on any step: Maximum of 2 attempts on each step
CS required at time of application: No

USCE Requirement: No
Cut-Off time since graduation: 5 years
Program offers couple match: Yes
Visas Sponsored or accepted: J1 visa and H1b visa

University of Chicago (NorthShore) Transitional Year Residency Program

Specialty: Transitional Year
Program name: University of Chicago (NorthShore) Program
Program code: 999-16-00-037
NRMP Code: 1160999P0
Program type: Community-based university affiliated hospital
State: Illinois
Address: Evanston Hospital,
          2650 Ridge Ave, Evanston, IL 60201
Phone: (847) 570-2509
Percentage of IMGs in the program: 0%
Minimum USMLE Step 1 Score Requirement: 220
Minimum USMLE Step 2 Score Requirement: 220
Attempts on any step: Must pass on first attempt including CS exam
CS required at time of application: No

USCE Requirement: Yes
Cut-Off time since graduation: 5 years unless clinically active as in residency or practice
Program offers couple match: Yes
Visas Sponsored or accepted: J1 visa and H1b visa

Swedish Covenant Hospital Transitional Year Residency Program

Specialty: Transitional Year
Program name: Swedish Covenant Hospital Program
Program code: 999-16-00-231
State: Illinois
Address: Swedish Covenant Hospital,
5145 N California Avenue, Chicago, Illinois 60625
Phone: (773) 989-3808
Percentage of IMGs in the program: 20%
Minimum USMLE Step 1 Score Requirement: No limits set
Minimum USMLE Step 2 Score Requirement: No limits set
Attempts on any step: No limits set
CS required at time of application: No
USCE Requirement: None
Cut-Off time since graduation: No limits set

Program offers couple match: Yes
Visas Sponsored or accepted: No visa

St. Joseph Hospital Transitional Year Residency Program

Specialty: Transitional Year
Program name: Presence St Joseph Hospital (Chicago) Program
Program code: 999-16-00-033
State: Illinois
Address: St Joseph Hospital,
            2900 N Lake Shore Dr, Chicago, IL 60657
Phone: (773) 665-3022
Fax: (773) 665-3384
Percentage of IMGs in the program: 0%
Minimum USMLE Step 1 Score Requirement: 205
Minimum USMLE Step 2 Score Requirement: 205
Attempts on any step: Maximum of 2 attempts on each step including CS exam
CS required at time of application: Yes including ECFMG certificate
USCE Requirement: None
Cut-Off time since graduation: 5 years unless clinically active as in residency of practice
Program offers couple match: Yes

Visas Sponsored or accepted: J1 visa and H1b visa

Presence Resurrection Medical Center Transitional Year Residency Program

Specialty: Transitional Year
Program name: Presence Resurrection Medical Center Program
Program code: 999-16-00-207
NRMP Code: 1937999P0
Program type: Community-based
State: Illinois
Address: Presence Resurrection Medical Center, 7435 W Talcott Ave, Chicago, IL 60631
Phone: (773) 990-5978
Fax: (773) 990-7635
Percentage of IMGs in the program: 0%
Minimum USMLE Step 1 Score Requirement: No limits set
Minimum USMLE Step 2 Score Requirement: No limits set
Attempts on any step: No limits set
CS required at time of application: Yes including ECFMG certificate
USCE Requirement: None
Cut-Off time since graduation: 5 years unless clinically active as in residency or practice

Program offers couple match: Yes
Visas Sponsored or accepted: No visa

Louis A Weiss Memorial Hospital Transitional Year Residency Program

Specialty: Transitional Year
Program name: Louis A Weiss Memorial Hospital Program
Program code: 999-16-00-035
NRMP Code: 1846999P0
Program type: Community-based university affiliated hospital
State: Illinois
Address: Louis A Weiss Memorial Hospital, Transitional Year Program,
4646 N Marine Dr, Chicago, IL 60640-9966
Phone: (773) 564-5225
Fax: (773) 564-5226
Percentage of IMGs in the program: 0%
Minimum USMLE Step 1 Score Requirement: 225
Minimum USMLE Step 2 Score Requirement: 225
Attempts on any step: No limits set
CS required at time of application: Yes
USCE Requirement: None

Cut-Off time since graduation: 3 years unless clinically active as in residency or practice
Program offers couple match: No
Visas Sponsored or accepted: J1 visa

MacNeal Hospital Transitional Year Residency Program

Specialty: Transitional Year
Program name: MacNeal Hospital Program
Program code: 999-16-00-032
NRMP Code: 1121999P0
Program type: Community-based university affiliated hospital
State: Illinois
Address: MacNeal Hospital,
          3249 S Oak Park Ave, Berwyn, IL 60402
Phone: (708) 783-3403
Fax: (708) 783-3341
Percentage of IMGs in the program: 0%
Minimum USMLE Step 1 Score Requirement: 235
Minimum USMLE Step 2 Score Requirement: 240
Attempts on any step: Must pass on first attempt on any step
CS required at time of application: Yes including ECFMG certificate

USCE Requirement: None
Cut-Off time since graduation: 3 years
Program offers couple match: No
Visas Sponsored or accepted: No visa

Indiana

Indiana University Health Ball Memorial Hospital Transitional Year Residency Program

Specialty: Transitional Year
Program name: Indiana University Health Ball Memorial Hospital Program
Program code: 999-17-00-157
NRMP Code: 1192999P0
Program type: Community-based
State: Indiana
Address: IU Health Ball Memorial Hospital, 2401 W University Ave, Muncie, IN 47303
Phone: (765) 741-1095
Fax: (765) 751-1451
Percentage of IMGs in the program: 0%
Minimum USMLE Step 1 Score Requirement: No limits set

Minimum USMLE Step 2 Score Requirement: No limits set
Attempts on any step: Must pass on first attempt
CS required at time of application: No
USCE Requirement: None
Cut-Off time since graduation: No limits set
Program offers couple match: Yes
Visas Sponsored or accepted: J1 visa and H1b visa

St. Vincent Hospitals and Health Care Center Transitional Year Residency Program

Specialty: Transitional Year
Program name: St Vincent Hospitals and Health Care Center Program
Program code: 999-17-00-041
NRMP Code: 1189999P0
Program type: Community-based university affiliated hospital
State: Indiana
Address: St Vincent Hospital and Health Care Center,
           2001 W 86th St, Indianapolis, IN 46260
Phone: (317) 338-6399
Fax: (317) 338-6359
Percentage of IMGs in the program: 0%

Minimum USMLE Step 1 Score Requirement:
No limits set
Minimum USMLE Step 2 Score Requirement:
No limits set
Attempts on any step: Must pass on first attempt including CS exam
CS required at time of application: Yes including ECFMG certificate
USCE Requirement: None
Cut-Off time since graduation: 3 years
Program offers couple match: Yes
Visas Sponsored or accepted: J1 visa

Indiana University School of Medicine/Methodist Hospital Transitional Year Residency Program

Specialty: Transitional Year
Program name: Indiana University School of Medicine/Methodist Hospital Program
Program code: 999-17-00-040
NRMP Code: 1187999P0
Program type: Community-based university affiliated hospital
State: Indiana
Address: IU Health Methodist Hospital,
          1633 N Capitol Ave, Indianapolis, IN 46202
Phone: (317) 962-8881

Fax: (317) 962-0838
Percentage of IMGs in the program: 0%
Minimum USMLE Step 1 Score Requirement: 220
Minimum USMLE Step 2 Score Requirement: 220
Attempts on any step: Must pass on first attempt including CS exam
CS required at time of application: Yes including ECFMG certificate
USCE Requirement: Yes
Cut-Off time since graduation: 3 years
Program offers couple match: Yes
Visas Sponsored or accepted: J1 visa

Iowa

Central Iowa Health System (Iowa Methodist Medical Center) Transitional Year Residency Program

Specialty: Transitional Year
Program name: Central Iowa Health System (Iowa Methodist Medical Center) Program
Program code: 999-18-00-220
NRMP Code: 1201999P0

Program type: Community-based university affiliated hospital
State: Iowa
Address: Iowa Methodist Medical Center,
         1415 Woodland Ave, Des Moines, IA 50309-9976
Phone: (515) 241-8595
Fax: (515) 241-4080
Percentage of IMGs in the program: 0%
Minimum USMLE Step 1 Score Requirement: 210
Minimum USMLE Step 2 Score Requirement: 210
Attempts on any step: No limits set
CS required at time of application: No
USCE Requirement: None
Cut-Off time since graduation: 3 years
Program offers couple match: No
Visas Sponsored or accepted: J1 visa

Broadlawns Medical Center Transitional Year Residency Program

Specialty: Transitional Year
Program name: Broadlawns Medical Center Program
Program code: 999-18-00-042
NRMP Code: 1199999P0

Program type: Community-based university affiliated hospital
State: Iowa
Address: Broadlawns Medical Center,
1801 Hickman Rd, Des Moines, IA 50314
Phone: (515) 282-2293
Fax: (515) 282-8193
Percentage of IMGs in the program: 0%
Minimum USMLE Step 1 Score Requirement: No limits set
Minimum USMLE Step 2 Score Requirement: No limits set
Attempts on any step: Maximum of 3 attempts on each step including CS exam
CS required at time of application: No
USCE Requirement: Yes
Cut-Off time since graduation: 5 years
Program offers couple match: No
Visas Sponsored or accepted: J1 visa

Maryland

Maryland General Hospital Transitional Year Residency Program

Specialty: Transitional Year

Program name: University of Maryland Medical Center Midtown Campus Program
Program code: 999-23-00-049
State: Maryland
Address: Maryland General Hospital,
827 Linden Ave, Baltimore, MD 21201
Phone: (410) 225-8790
Fax: (410) 225-8910
Percentage of IMGs in the program: 80%
Minimum USMLE Step 1 Score Requirement: 205
Minimum USMLE Step 2 Score Requirement: 205
Attempts on any step: Must pass on first attempt
CS required at time of application: No
USCE Requirement: None
Cut-Off time since graduation: 5 years
Program offers couple match: No
Visas Sponsored or accepted: J1 visa

Harbor Hospital Center Transitional Year Residency Program

Specialty: Transitional Year
Program name: Harbor Hospital Center Program
Program code: 999-23-00-050
NRMP Code: 1250999P0

Program type: Community-based
State: Maryland
Address: MedStar Harbor Hospital,
           3001 S Hanover St, Baltimore, MD 21225
Phone: (410) 350-3565
Fax: (410) 354-0186
Percentage of IMGs in the program: 50%
Minimum USMLE Step 1 Score Requirement: 230
Minimum USMLE Step 2 Score Requirement: 230
Attempts on any step: Must pass on first attempt
CS required at time of application: No
USCE Requirement: None
Cut-Off time since graduation: No limits set
Program offers couple match: Yes
Visas Sponsored or accepted: J1 visa

Massachusetts

Newton-Wellesley Hospital Transitional Year Residency Program

Specialty: Transitional Year

Program name: Newton-Wellesley Hospital Program
Program code: 999-24-00-246
NRMP Code: 1280999P0
Program type: Community-based university affiliated hospital
State: Massachusetts
Address: Newton-Wellesley Hospital,
          2014 Washington St, Newton Lower Falls, MA 02462
Phone: (617) 243-6467
Fax: (617) 243-6701
Percentage of IMGs in the program: 0%
Minimum USMLE Step 1 Score Requirement: 230
Minimum USMLE Step 2 Score Requirement: 230
Attempts on any step: Must pass on first attempt including CS exam
CS required at time of application: Yes
USCE Requirement: None
Cut-Off time since graduation: 2 years
Program offers couple match: No
Visas Sponsored or accepted: No visa

Tufts Medical Center/Lemuel Shattuck Hospital Transitional Year Residency Program

Specialty: Transitional Year

Program name: Tufts Medical Center/Lemuel Shattuck Hospital Program
Program code: 999-24-00-199
State: Massachusetts
Address: Lemuel Shattuck Hospital,
            170 Morton St, Jamaica Plain, MA 02130-3782
Phone: (617) 971-3337
Fax: (617) 971-3852
Percentage of IMGs in the program: 0%
Minimum USMLE Step 1 Score Requirement: 220
Minimum USMLE Step 2 Score Requirement: 220
Attempts on any step: Must pass on first attempt including CS exam
CS required at time of application: No
USCE Requirement: 3 months
Cut-Off time since graduation: 3 years
Program offers couple match: Yes
Visas Sponsored or accepted: J1 visa

MetroWest Medical Center/Harvard Medical School Transitional Year Residency Program

Specialty: Transitional Year

Program name: MetroWest Medical Center/Harvard Medical School Program
Program code: 999-24-00-160
NRMP Code: 1812999P0
Program type: Community-based university affiliated hospital
State: Massachusetts
Address: MetroWest Medical Center,
        115 Lincoln St, Framingham, MA 01702
Phone: (508) 383-1555
Fax: (508) 872-4794
Percentage of IMGs in the program: 50%
Minimum USMLE Step 1 Score Requirement: 205
Minimum USMLE Step 2 Score Requirement: 205
Attempts on any step: No limits set
CS required at time of application: No
USCE Requirement: None
Cut-Off time since graduation: 5 years unless clinically active as in residency or practice
Program offers couple match: Yes
Visas Sponsored or accepted: J1 visa

Cambridge Health Alliance Transitional Year Residency Program

Specialty: Transitional Year

Program name: Cambridge Health Alliance Program
Program code: 999-24-00-054
NRMP Code: 1268999P0
Program type: Community-based university affiliated hospital
State: Massachusetts
Address: Cambridge Hospital,
          1493 Cambridge St, Cambridge, MA 02139
Phone: (617) 665-1021
Fax: (617) 665-2151
Percentage of IMGs in the program: 0%
Minimum USMLE Step 1 Score Requirement: No limits set
Minimum USMLE Step 2 Score Requirement: No limits set
Attempts on any step: No limits set
CS required at time of application: No
USCE Requirement: Yes 1 month
Cut-Off time since graduation: No limits set
Program offers couple match: Yes
Visas Sponsored or accepted: J1 visa

Tufts Medical Center Transitional Year Residency Program

Specialty: Transitional Year
Program name: Tufts Medical Center Program
Program code: 999-24-00-158

NRMP Code: 1263999P0
Program type: Community-based university affiliated hospital
State: Massachusetts
Address: Signature Healthcare Brockton Hospital, Transitional Year Program,
        680 Centre St, Brockton, MA 02302
Phone: (508) 941-7210
Fax: (508) 941-6336
Percentage of IMGs in the program: 0%
Minimum USMLE Step 1 Score Requirement: 210
Minimum USMLE Step 2 Score Requirement: 210
Attempts on any step: No limits set
CS required at time of application: Yes including ECFMG certificate
USCE Requirement: None
Cut-Off time since graduation: 2 years
Program offers couple match: Yes
Visas Sponsored or accepted: No visa

Steward Carney Hospital Transitional Year Residency Program

Specialty: Transitional Year
Program name: Steward Carney Hospital Program
Program code: 999-24-00-159

NRMP Code: 1258999P0
Program type: Community-based university affiliated hospital
State: Massachusetts
Address: Carney Hospital,
2100 Dorchester Ave, Boston, MA 02124-5666
Phone: (617) 506-2726
Fax: (617) 506-2110
Percentage of IMGs in the program: 0%
Minimum USMLE Step 1 Score Requirement: 210
Minimum USMLE Step 2 Score Requirement: 210
Attempts on any step: Must pass on first attempt
CS required at time of application: No
USCE Requirement: None
Cut-Off time since graduation: No limits set
Program offers couple match: Yes
Visas Sponsored or accepted: J1 visa

Michigan

Oakwood Heritage Hospital Transitional Year Residency Program

Specialty: Transitional Year
Program name: Oakwood Heritage Hospital Program
Program code: 999-25-00-258
Program type: Community-based university affiliated hospital
State: Michigan
Address: Oakwood Heritage Hospital, 18101 Oakwood Blvd, Dearborn, MI 48124
Phone: (313) 436-2581
Fax: (313) 436-2071
Percentage of IMGs in the program: 15%
Minimum USMLE Step 1 Score Requirement: 210
Minimum USMLE Step 2 Score Requirement: 210
Attempts on any step: Must pass on first attempt
CS required at time of application: No
USCE Requirement: Yes
Cut-Off time since graduation: 5 years
Program offers couple match: No
Visas Sponsored or accepted: No visa

St. Mary Mercy Hospital Transitional Year Residency Program

Specialty: Transitional Year
Program name: St Mary Mercy Hospital Program
Program code: 999-25-00-255
NRMP Code: 1418999P0
Program type: Community-based
State: Michigan
Address: St Mary Mercy Hospital,
      36475 Five Mile Rd, Livonia, MI 48154
Phone: (734) 655-2704
Fax: (734) 655-8430
Percentage of IMGs in the program: 25%
Minimum USMLE Step 1 Score Requirement: No limits set
Minimum USMLE Step 2 Score Requirement: No limits set
Attempts on any step: Must pass on first attempt
CS required at time of application: No
USCE Requirement: None
Cut-Off time since graduation: 3 years
Program offers couple match: Yes
Visas Sponsored or accepted: J1 visa

Wayne State University School of Medicine Transitional Year Residency Program

Specialty: Transitional Year
Program name: Wayne State University School of Medicine Program
Program code: 999-25-00-253
NRMP Code: 1361999P0
Program type: University-based
State: Michigan
Address: Crittenton Hospital Medical Center, 1101 W University Dr, Rochester, MI 48307
Phone: (248) 601-4900
Fax: (248) 601-4994
Percentage of IMGs in the program: 15%
Minimum USMLE Step 1 Score Requirement: 205
Minimum USMLE Step 2 Score Requirement: 205
Attempts on any step: Must pass on first attempt including CS exam
CS required at time of application: No
USCE Requirement: 6 months
Cut-Off time since graduation: 5 years
Program offers couple match: Yes
Visas Sponsored or accepted: J1 visa

Providence Hospital and Medical Centers Transitional Year Residency Program

Specialty: Transitional Year
Program name: Providence Hospital and Medical Centers Program
Program code: 999-25-00-068
NRMP Code: 1303999P1, 1303999P0
Program type: Community-based
State: Michigan
Address: Providence Hospital and Medical Center,
          16001 W Nine Mile Rd, Southfield, MI 48075
Phone: (248) 849-8441
Fax: (248) 849-5324
Percentage of IMGs in the program: 40%
Minimum USMLE Step 1 Score Requirement: 220
Minimum USMLE Step 2 Score Requirement: 220
Attempts on any step: Must pass on first attempt including CS exam
CS required at time of application: Yes including ECFMG certificate
USCE Requirement: None
Cut-Off time since graduation: 3 years
Program offers couple match: Yes
Visas Sponsored or accepted: J1 visa and H1b visa

St. Joseph Mercy-Oakland Transitional Year Residency Program

Specialty: Transitional Year
Program name: St Joseph Mercy-Oakland Program
Program code: 999-25-00-067
NRMP Code: 1319999P0
Program type: Community-based university affiliated hospital
State: Michigan
Address: St Joseph Mercy Oakland,
          44405 Woodward Ave, Pontiac, MI 48341
Phone: (248) 858-6233
Fax: (248) 858-3244
Percentage of IMGs in the program: 70%
Minimum USMLE Step 1 Score Requirement: 210
Minimum USMLE Step 2 Score Requirement: 210
Attempts on any step: Must pass on first attempt
CS required at time of application: No
USCE Requirement: None
Cut-Off time since graduation: 3 years
Program offers couple match: Yes
Visas Sponsored or accepted: J1 visa

Western Michigan University School of Medicine Transitional Year Residency Program

Specialty: Transitional Year
Program name: Western Michigan University School of Medicine Program
Program code: 999-25-00-065
NRMP Code: 1314999P0
Program type: Community-based university affiliated hospital
State: Michigan
Address: Western Michigan University School of Medicine,
       1000 Oakland Dr, Kalamazoo, MI 49008-1284
Phone: (269) 337-6353
Fax: (269) 337-4262
Percentage of IMGs in the program: 0%
Minimum USMLE Step 1 Score Requirement: 225
Minimum USMLE Step 2 Score Requirement: 225
Attempts on any step: No limits set
CS required at time of application: No
USCE Requirement: None
Cut-Off time since graduation: 5 years
Program offers couple match: Yes

Visas Sponsored or accepted: J1 visa and H1b visa

St. John Hospital and Medical Center Transitional Year Residency Program

Specialty: Transitional Year
Program name: St John Hospital and Medical Center Program
Program code: 999-25-00-059
NRMP Code: 1915999P0
Program type: Community-based university affiliated hospital
State: Michigan
Address: St John Hospital and Medical Center, 22101 Moross Rd, Detroit, MI 48236
Phone: (313) 343-3875
Fax: (313) 343-7840
Percentage of IMGs in the program: 0%
Minimum USMLE Step 1 Score Requirement: 205
Minimum USMLE Step 2 Score Requirement: 205
Attempts on any step: Must pass on first attempt
CS required at time of application: No
USCE Requirement: None
Cut-Off time since graduation: 5 years unless clinically active as in residency or practice

Program offers couple match: Yes
Visas Sponsored or accepted: J1 visa

Grand Rapids Medical Education Partners/Michigan State University Transitional Year Residency Program

Specialty: Transitional Year
Program name: Grand Rapids Medical Education Partners/Michigan State University Program
Program code: 999-25-00-190
NRMP Code: 2077999P0
Program type: Community-based
State: Michigan
Address: Grand Rapids Medical Education Partners,
           25 Michigan Ave NE, Grand Rapids, MI 49503
Phone: (616) 391-3245
Fax: (616) 391-3130
Percentage of IMGs in the program: 10%
Minimum USMLE Step 1 Score Requirement: No limits set
Minimum USMLE Step 2 Score Requirement: No limits set
Attempts on any step: No limits set
CS required at time of application: No

USCE Requirement: Yes
Cut-Off time since graduation: 3 years
Program offers couple match: Yes
Visas Sponsored or accepted: J1 visa

Hurley Medical Center/Michigan State University Transitional Year Residency Program

Specialty: Transitional Year
Program name: Hurley Medical Center/Michigan State University Program
Program code: 999-25-00-062
NRMP Code: 1307999P1, 1307999P0
Program type: Community-based university affiliated hospital
State: Michigan
Address: Hurley Med Center,
          Two Hurley Plaza, Flint, MI 48503
Phone: (810) 262-9080
Fax: (810) 262-7245
Percentage of IMGs in the program: 50%
Minimum USMLE Step 1 Score Requirement: 213
Minimum USMLE Step 2 Score Requirement: 213
Attempts on any step: Maximum of 2 attempts on any step including CS exam
CS required at time of application: No
USCE Requirement: None

Cut-Off time since graduation: 5 years
Program offers couple match: Yes
Visas Sponsored or accepted: J1 visa and H1b visa

Detroit Medical Center/Wayne State University (Sinai-Grace) Transitional Year Residency Program

Specialty: Transitional Year
Program name: Detroit Medical Center/Wayne State University (Sinai-Grace) Program
Program code: 999-25-00-060
NRMP Code: 1374999P0, 1374999P1
Program type: University-based
State: Michigan
Address: Sinai-Grace Hospital,
        6071 W Outer Dr, Detroit, MI 48235
Phone: (313) 966-3189
Fax: (313) 966-1738
Percentage of IMGs in the program: 80%
Minimum USMLE Step 1 Score Requirement: 200
Minimum USMLE Step 2 Score Requirement: 205
Attempts on any step: Must pass on first attempt
CS required at time of application: No
USCE Requirement: None

Cut-Off time since graduation: 3 years unless clinically active as in residency or practice
Program offers couple match: Yes
Visas Sponsored or accepted: J1 visa

Henry Ford Hospital/Wayne State University Transitional Year Residency Program

Specialty: Transitional Year
Program name: Henry Ford Hospital/Wayne State University Program
Program code: 999-25-00-058
NRMP Code: 1300999P0, 1300999P2
Program type: Community-based university affiliated hospital
State: Michigan
Address: Henry Ford Hospital,
             2799 W Grand Blvd, Detroit, MI 48202
Phone: (313) 916-2889
Fax: (313) 916-1394
Percentage of IMGs in the program: 0%
Minimum USMLE Step 1 Score Requirement: 225
Minimum USMLE Step 2 Score Requirement: 225
Attempts on any step: Must pass on first attempt
CS required at time of application: No
USCE Requirement: No

Cut-Off time since graduation: 4 years
Program offers couple match: Yes
Visas Sponsored or accepted: J1 visa

Oakwood Hospital Transitional Year Residency Program

Specialty: Transitional Year
Program name: Oakwood Hospital Program
Program code: 999-25-00-057
NRMP Code: 1946999P0
Program type: Community-based university affiliated hospital
State: Michigan
Address: Oakwood Hospital and Medical Center,

18101 Oakwood Blvd, Dearborn, MI 48124
Phone: (313) 436-2581
Fax: (313) 436-2071
Percentage of IMGs in the program: 0%
Minimum USMLE Step 1 Score Requirement: 230
Minimum USMLE Step 2 Score Requirement: 230
Attempts on any step: Must pass on first attempt
CS required at time of application: No
USCE Requirement: Yes
Cut-Off time since graduation: 3 years

Program offers couple match: No
Visas Sponsored or accepted: No visa

St. Joseph Mercy Hospital Transitional Year Residency Program

Specialty: Transitional Year
Program name: St Joseph Mercy Hospital Program
Program code: 999-25-00-056
 Program type: Community-based university affiliated hospital
State: Michigan
Address: St Joseph Mercy Hospital,
          5333 McAuley Dr, Ann Arbor, MI 48106
Phone: (734) 712-5563
Fax: (734) 712-5583
Percentage of IMGs in the program: 0%
Minimum USMLE Step 1 Score Requirement: 210
Minimum USMLE Step 2 Score Requirement: 210
Attempts on any step: Must pass on first attempt
CS required at time of application: No
USCE Requirement: None

Cut-Off time since graduation: 2 years
Program offers couple match: Yes
Visas Sponsored or accepted: J1 visa

Minnesota

Hennepin County Medical Center Transitional Year Residency Program

Specialty: Transitional Year
Program name: Hennepin County Medical Center Program
Program code: 999-26-00-069
 State: Minnesota
Address: Hennepin County Medical Center, 701 Park Ave S, Minneapolis, MN 55415-1829
Phone: (612) 873-3922
Fax: (612) 904-4401
Percentage of IMGs in the program: 10%
Minimum USMLE Step 1 Score Requirement: No limits set
Minimum USMLE Step 2 Score Requirement: No limits set
Attempts on any step: No limits set
CS required at time of application: No

USCE Requirement: None
Cut-Off time since graduation: No limits set
Program offers couple match: Yes
Visas Sponsored or accepted: No visa

Missouri

Mercy Hospital (St Louis) Transitional Year Residency Program

Specialty: Transitional Year
Program name: Mercy Hospital (St Louis) Program
Program code: 999-28-00-071
NRMP Code: 1362999P0
Program type: Community-based university affiliated hospital
State: Missouri
Address: Mercy Hospital St Louis,
          615 S New Ballas Rd, St Louis, MO 63141-8277
Phone: (314) 251-6930
Fax: (314) 251-4288
Percentage of IMGs in the program: 0%
Minimum USMLE Step 1 Score Requirement: 220

Minimum USMLE Step 2 Score Requirement: 220
Attempts on any step: Must pass on first attempt
CS required at time of application: Yes including CS exam
USCE Requirement: None
Cut-Off time since graduation: 2 years
Program offers couple match: Yes
Visas Sponsored or accepted: No visa

New York

Lincoln Medical and Mental Health Center Transitional Year Residency Program

Specialty: Transitional Year
Program name: Lincoln Medical and Mental Health Center Program
Program code: 999-35-00-257
 State: New York
Address: Lincoln Medical and Mental Health Center,
        234 E 149th St, Bronx, NY 10451

Phone: (718) 579-5000
Fax: (718) 579-5246
Percentage of IMGs in the program: 30%
Minimum USMLE Step 1 Score Requirement: 210
Minimum USMLE Step 2 Score Requirement: 210
Attempts on any step: Must pass in first attempt
CS required at time of application: No
USCE Requirement: None
Cut-Off time since graduation: No limits set
Program offers couple match: Yes
Visas Sponsored or accepted: J1 visa and H1b visa

St. Joseph Hospital Health Center Transitional Year Residency Program

Specialty: Transitional Year
Program name: St Joseph's Hospital Health Center Program
Program code: 999-35-00-084
NRMP Code: 1518999P0
Program type: Community-based university affiliated hospital
State: New York
Address: St Joseph's Hospital Health Center, 301 Prospect Ave, Syracuse, NY 13203

Phone: (315) 448-5547
Fax: (315) 448-6313
Percentage of IMGs in the program: 0%
Minimum USMLE Step 1 Score Requirement: 210
Minimum USMLE Step 2 Score Requirement: 210
Attempts on any step: Must pass on first attempt including CS exam
CS required at time of application: Yes
USCE Requirement: Yes
Cut-Off time since graduation: 5 years
Program offers couple match: Yes
Visas Sponsored or accepted: No visa

Memorial Sloan-Kettering Cancer Center Transitional Year Residency Program

Specialty: Transitional Year
Program name: Memorial Sloan-Kettering Cancer Center Program
Program code: 999-35-00-241
State: New York
Address: Memorial Sloan-Kettering Cancer Center,
    1275 York Ave, New York, NY 10021
Phone: (212) 639-3210
Fax: (646) 422-2135
Percentage of IMGs in the program: 0%

Minimum USMLE Step 1 Score Requirement: No limits set
Minimum USMLE Step 2 Score Requirement: No limits set
Attempts on any step: No limits set
CS required at time of application: No
USCE Requirement: None
Cut-Off time since graduation: No limits set
Program offers couple match: Yes
Visas Sponsored or accepted: J1 visa

New York Medical College (Sound Shore) Transitional Year Residency Program

Specialty: Transitional Year
Program name: New York Medical College (Sound Shore) Program
Program code: 999-35-00-216
State: New York
Address: Sound Shore Medical Center Westchester,
        16 Guion Pl, New Rochelle, NY 10802
Phone: (914) 365-3681
Fax: (914) 365-5489
Percentage of IMGs in the program: 20%
Minimum USMLE Step 1 Score Requirement: 205
Minimum USMLE Step 2 Score Requirement: 205

Attempts on any step: Must pass on first attempt
CS required at time of application: No
USCE Requirement: None
Cut-Off time since graduation: 10 years
Program offers couple match: Yes
Visas Sponsored or accepted: J1 visa and H1b visa

United Health Services Hospitals Transitional Year Residency Program

Specialty: Transitional Year
Program name: United Health Services Hospitals Program
Program code: 999-35-00-081
NRMP Code: 1452999P0
Program type: Community-based university affiliated hospital
State: New York
Address: UHS Wilson Medical Center,
          33-57 Harrison St, Johnson City, NY 13790
Phone: (800) 338-8471
Fax: (607) 798-1629
Percentage of IMGs in the program: 15%
Minimum USMLE Step 1 Score Requirement: 210

Minimum USMLE Step 2 Score Requirement: 210
Attempts on any step: No limits set
CS required at time of application: No
USCE Requirement: None
Cut-Off time since graduation: No limits set
Program offers couple match: Yes
Visas Sponsored or accepted: J1 visa and H1b visa

New York Hospital Medical Center of Queens/Cornell University Medical College Transitional Year Residency Program

Specialty: Transitional Year
Program name: New York Hospital Medical Center of Queens/Cornell University Medical College Program
Program code: 999-35-00-225
 State: New York
Address: New York Hospital Queens,
           56-45 Main St, Flushing, NY 11355
Phone: (718) 670-1477
Fax: (718) 460-1352
Percentage of IMGs in the program: 0%
Minimum USMLE Step 1 Score Requirement: 210
Minimum USMLE Step 2 Score Requirement: 210

Attempts on any step: Must pass on first attempt
CS required at time of application: No
USCE Requirement: None
Cut-Off time since graduation: No limits set
Program offers couple match: No
Visas Sponsored or accepted: J1 visa and H1b visa

Bassett Medical Center Transitional Year Residency Program

Specialty: Transitional Year
Program name: Bassett Medical Center Program
Program code: 999-35-00-080
NRMP Code: 1442999P0, 1442999P1
Program type: Community-based university affiliated hospital
State: New York
Address: Mary Imogene Bassett Hospital, One Atwell Rd, Cooperstown, NY 13326
Phone: (607) 547-3764
Fax: (607) 547-6612
Percentage of IMGs in the program: 0%
Minimum USMLE Step 1 Score Requirement: 205
Minimum USMLE Step 2 Score Requirement: 204

Attempts on any step: Must pass on first attempt including CS exam
CS required at time of application: Yes including ECFMG certificate
USCE Requirement: None
Cut-Off time since graduation: 5 years
Program offers couple match: Yes
Visas Sponsored or accepted: J1 visa and H1b visa

North Dakota

University of North Dakota Transitional Year Residency Program

Specialty: Transitional Year
Program name: University of North Dakota Program
Program code: 999-37-00-086
NRMP Code: 1539999P0
Program type: Community-based university affiliated hospital
State: North Dakota
Address: Sanford Health,
        801 Broadway N, Fargo, ND 58122-0170
Phone: (701) 234-5934

Fax: (701) 234-7230
Percentage of IMGs in the program: 0%
Minimum USMLE Step 1 Score Requirement:
No limits set
Minimum USMLE Step 2 Score Requirement:
No limits set
Attempts on any step: Must pass on first
attempt
CS required at time of application: Yes
including ECFMG certificate
USCE Requirement: No
Cut-Off time since graduation: 3 years
Program offers couple match: No
Visas Sponsored or accepted: No visa

Ohio

Akron General Medical Center/NEOMED Transitional Year Residency Program

Specialty: Transitional Year
Program name: Akron General Medical
Center/NEOMED Program
Program code: 999-38-00-088
NRMP Code: 1542999P0
Program type: Community-based university
affiliated hospital

State: Ohio
Address: Akron General Medical Center,
           400 Wabash Ave, Akron, OH 44307
Phone: (330) 344-6140
Fax: (330) 535-9270
Percentage of IMGs in the program: 0%
Minimum USMLE Step 1 Score Requirement:
220
Minimum USMLE Step 2 Score Requirement:
220
Attempts on any step: No limits set
CS required at time of application: No
USCE Requirement: None
Cut-Off time since graduation: 5 years
Program offers couple match: Yes
Visas Sponsored or accepted: J1 visa and H1b
visa

Summa Health System/NEOMED Transitional Year Residency Program

Specialty: Transitional Year
Program name: Summa Health
System/NEOMED Program
Program code: 999-38-00-087
NRMP Code: 1541999P0
Program type: Community-based university
affiliated hospital
State: Ohio

Address: Summa Health System, Transitional Year Program,
    525 E Market St, Akron, OH 44309
Phone: (330) 375-3202
Fax: (330) 375-3760
Percentage of IMGs in the program: 0%
Minimum USMLE Step 1 Score Requirement: 210
Minimum USMLE Step 2 Score Requirement: 210
Attempts on any step: Must pass on first attempt
CS required at time of application: Yes
USCE Requirement: None
Cut-Off time since graduation: 3 years
Program offers couple match: Yes
Visas Sponsored or accepted: J1 visa

Aultman Hospital/NEOMED Transitional Year Residency Program

Specialty: Transitional Year
Program name: Aultman Hospital/NEOMED Program
Program code: 999-38-00-191
State: Ohio
Address: 2600 sixth ST SW, Canton, OH 44710-1799
Phone: (330) 363-6293

Percentage of IMGs in the program: 0%
Minimum USMLE Step 1 Score Requirement: 210
Minimum USMLE Step 2 Score Requirement: 210
Attempts on any step: Must pass on first attempt
CS required at time of application: No
USCE Requirement: Yes
Cut-Off time since graduation: 2 years
Program offers couple match: Yes
Visas Sponsored or accepted: J1 visa and H1b visa

Mount Carmel Health System Transitional Year Residency Program

Specialty: Transitional Year
Program name: Mount Carmel Health System Program
Program code: 999-38-00-093
State: Ohio
Address: Mount Carmel Health System,
            793 W State St, Columbus, OH 43222
Phone: (614) 234-1444 or (614) 234-1079
Fax: (614) 234-2772
Percentage of IMGs in the program: 25% (not every year they have IMGs)

Minimum USMLE Step 1 Score Requirement: 210
Minimum USMLE Step 2 Score Requirement: 210
Attempts on any step: Must pass on first attempt
CS required at time of application: Yes including ECFMG certificate
USCE Requirement: Yes
Cut-Off time since graduation: 5 years
Program offers couple match: Yes
Visas Sponsored or accepted: No visa

Riverside Methodist Hospitals (OhioHealth) Transitional Year Residency Program

Specialty: Transitional Year
Program name: Riverside Methodist Hospitals (OhioHealth) Program
Program code: 999-38-00-095
NRMP Code: 1567999P0
Program type: Community-based
State: Ohio
Address: Riverside Methodist Hospital,
          3535 Olentangy River Rd, Columbus, OH 43214-3998
Phone: (614) 566-5468
Fax: (614) 566-1073
Percentage of IMGs in the program: 0%

Minimum USMLE Step 1 Score Requirement: No limits set
Minimum USMLE Step 2 Score Requirement: No limits set
Attempts on any step: No limits set
CS required at time of application: Yes
USCE Requirement: None
Cut-Off time since graduation: 2 years unless clinically active as in residency or practice
Program offers couple match: Yes
Visas Sponsored or accepted: J1 visa

Kettering Medical Center Transitional Year Residency Program

Specialty: Transitional Year
Program name: Kettering Medical Center Program
Program code: 999-38-00-096
NRMP Code: 1576999P0
Program type: Community-based university affiliated hospital
State: Ohio
Address: Kettering Medical Center,
          3535 Southern Blvd, Kettering, OH 45429
Phone: (937) 395-8609 and (800) 203-8925
Fax: (937) 395-8023
Percentage of IMGs in the program: 0%

Minimum USMLE Step 1 Score Requirement: 225

Minimum USMLE Step 2 Score Requirement: 225

Attempts on any step: Must pass on first attempt

CS required at time of application: No

USCE Requirement: Yes

Cut-Off time since graduation: 5 years

Program offers couple match: Yes

Visas Sponsored or accepted: J1 visa

Mercy St Vincent Medical Center/Mercy Health Partners Transitional Year Residency Program

Specialty: Transitional Year

Program name: Mercy St Vincent Medical Center/Mercy Health Partners Program

Program code: 999-38-00-165

NRMP Code: 1580999P0

Program type: Community-based university affiliated hospital

State: Ohio

Address: Mercy St Vincent Medical Center, 2200 Jefferson Ave, Toledo, OH 43604

Phone: (419) 251-1395

Fax: (419) 242-9806

Percentage of IMGs in the program: 0%

Minimum USMLE Step 1 Score Requirement: 203
Minimum USMLE Step 2 Score Requirement: 210
Attempts on any step: Must pass on first attempt
CS required at time of application: Yes
USCE Requirement: None
Cut-Off time since graduation: 5 years
Program offers couple match: Yes
Visas Sponsored or accepted: J1 visa and H1b visa

St. Elizabeth Health Center Transitional Year Residency Program

Specialty: Transitional Year
Program name: St Elizabeth Health Center Program
Program code: 999-38-00-250
NRMP Code: 1584999P0
Program type: Community-based university affiliated hospital
State: Ohio
Address: St Elizabeth Health Center,
         1044 Belmont Ave, Youngstown, OH 44501
Phone: (330) 480-2994
Fax: (330) 480-6601

Percentage of IMGs in the program: 0%
Minimum USMLE Step 1 Score Requirement: 206
Minimum USMLE Step 2 Score Requirement: 206
Attempts on any step: Maximum of 2 attempts allowed on each step
CS required at time of application: Yes including ECFMG certificate
USCE Requirement: None
Cut-Off time since graduation: 3 years
Program offers couple match: Yes
Visas Sponsored or accepted: J1 visa

Oregon

Legacy Emanuel Hospital and Health Center Transitional Year Residency Program

Specialty: Transitional Year
Program name: Legacy Emanuel Hospital and Health Center Program
Program code: 999-40-00-101
NRMP Code: Legacy Emanuel Hospital and Health Center, Transitional Year Program,

2801 N Gantenbein Ave, Portland, OR 97227

State: Oregon

Address: Legacy Emanuel Hospital and Health Center, Transitional Year Program, 2801 N Gantenbein Ave, Portland, OR 97227

Phone: (503) 413-4692

Fax: (503) 413-2980

Percentage of IMGs in the program: 0%

Minimum USMLE Step 1 Score Requirement: 210

Minimum USMLE Step 2 Score Requirement: 210

Attempts on any step: Must pass on first attempt including CS exam

CS required at time of application: No

USCE Requirement: Yes 3 months

Cut-Off time since graduation: 5 years

Program offers couple match: Yes

Visas Sponsored or accepted: No visa

Pennsylvania

Lehigh Valley Health Network/University of South Florida College of Medicine Transitional Year Residency Program

Specialty: Transitional Year
Program name: Lehigh Valley Health Network/University of South Florida College of Medicine Program
Program code: 999-41-00-103
NRMP Code: 1601999P0
Program type: Community-based university affiliated hospital
State: Pennsylvania
Address: Lehigh Valley Health Network,
          1240 S Cedar Crest Blvd, Allentown, PA 18103
Phone: (610) 402-4412
Fax: (610) 402-1675
Percentage of IMGs in the program: 0%
Minimum USMLE Step 1 Score Requirement: 210
Minimum USMLE Step 2 Score Requirement: 210
Attempts on any step: Must pass on first attempt including CS exam
CS required at time of application: No
USCE Requirement: None
Cut-Off time since graduation: 5 years

Program offers couple match: Yes
Visas Sponsored or accepted: J1 visa and H1b visa

St. Luke Hospital Transitional Year Residency Program

Specialty: Transitional Year
Program name: St Luke's Hospital Program
Program code: 999-41-00-104
NRMP Code: 1605999P0
Program type: University-based
State: Pennsylvania
Address: St Luke's University Hospital,
          801 Ostrum St, Bethlehem, PA 18015
Phone: (484) 526-4644
Fax: (484) 526-4920
Percentage of IMGs in the program: 0%
Minimum USMLE Step 1 Score Requirement:
No limits set
Minimum USMLE Step 2 Score Requirement:
No limits set
Attempts on any step: Must pass on first attempt
CS required at time of application: No
USCE Requirement: None
Cut-Off time since graduation: No limits set
Program offers couple match: No
Visas Sponsored or accepted: J1 visa and H1b visa

Mercy Catholic Medical Center Transitional Year Residency Program

Specialty: Transitional Year
Program name: Mercy Catholic Medical Center Program
Program code: 999-41-00-106
NRMP Code: 1636999P0
Program type: Community-based university affiliated hospital
State: Pennsylvania
Address: Mercy Catholic Medical Center, 1500 Lansdowne Ave, Darby, PA 19023
Phone: (610) 237-4685
Fax: (610) 237-5093
Percentage of IMGs in the program: 35%
Minimum USMLE Step 1 Score Requirement: No limits set
Minimum USMLE Step 2 Score Requirement: No limits set
Attempts on any step: No limits set
CS required at time of application: No
USCE Requirement: No
Cut-Off time since graduation: No limits set
Program offers couple match: Yes
Visas Sponsored or accepted: J1 visa and H1b visa

Albert Einstein Healthcare Network Transitional Year Residency Program

Specialty: Transitional Year
Program name: Albert Einstein Healthcare Network Program
Program code: 999-41-00-224
NRMP Code: 1631999P0, 1631999P1
Program type: Community-based university affiliated hospital
State: Pennsylvania
Address: Albert Einstein Medical Center,
5401 Old York Rd, Philadelphia, PA 19141-3025
Phone: (800) 220-2362
Fax: (215) 456-7926
Percentage of IMGs in the program: 0%
Minimum USMLE Step 1 Score Requirement: No limits set
Minimum USMLE Step 2 Score Requirement: No limits set
Attempts on any step: Must pass on first attempt
CS required at time of application: No
USCE Requirement: None
Cut-Off time since graduation: No limits set
Program offers couple match: Yes

Visas Sponsored or accepted: J1 visa and H1b visa

UPMC Medical Education (Mercy) Transitional Year Residency Program

Specialty: Transitional Year
Program name: UPMC Medical Education (Mercy) Program
Program code: 999-41-00-114
NRMP Code: 1649999P0
Program type: Community-based university affiliated hospital
State: Pennsylvania
Address: UPMC Mercy,
1400 Locust St, Pittsburgh, PA 15219-5166
Phone: (412) 232-8080
Fax: (412) 232-5689
Percentage of IMGs in the program: 0%
Minimum USMLE Step 1 Score Requirement: 220
Minimum USMLE Step 2 Score Requirement: 220
Attempts on any step: No limits set
CS required at time of application: No
USCE Requirement: None
Cut-Off time since graduation: No limits set
Program offers couple match: Yes

Visas Sponsored or accepted: None

UPMC Medical Education (Presbyterian Shadyside Hospital) Transitional Year Residency Program

Specialty: Transitional Year
Program name: UPMC Medical Education (Presbyterian Shadyside Hospital) Program
Program code: 999-41-00-117
State: Pennsylvania
Address: UPMC Presbyterian Shadyside,
5230 Centre Ave, Pittsburgh, PA 15232
Phone: (412) 623-2465
Fax: (412) 623-3592
Percentage of IMGs in the program: 35%
Minimum USMLE Step 1 Score Requirement: 204
Minimum USMLE Step 2 Score Requirement: 204
Attempts on any step: No limits set
CS required at time of application: Yes including ECFMG certificate
USCE Requirement: None
Cut-Off time since graduation: 2 years
Program offers couple match: Yes
Visas Sponsored or accepted: J1 visa and H1b visa

UPMC Medical Education Transitional Year Residency Program

Specialty: Transitional Year
Program name: UPMC Medical Education Program
Program code: 999-41-00-115
NRMP Code: 1652999P0, 1652999P1
Program type: University-based
State: Pennsylvania
Address: University of Pittsburgh Medical Center,
       200 Lothrop St, Pittsburgh, PA 15213
Phone: (412) 692-4945
Fax: (412) 692-4944
Percentage of IMGs in the program: 0%
Minimum USMLE Step 1 Score Requirement: No limits set
Minimum USMLE Step 2 Score Requirement: No limits set
Attempts on any step: No limits set
CS required at time of application: Yes
USCE Requirement: None
Cut-Off time since graduation: 5 years
Program offers couple match: Yes
Visas Sponsored or accepted: J1 visa and H1b visa

Crozer-Chester Medical Center Transitional Year Residency Program

Specialty: Transitional Year
Program name: Crozer-Chester Medical Center Program
Program code: 999-41-00-212
NRMP Code: 3185999P0
Program type: Community-based university affiliated hospital
State: Pennsylvania
Address: Crozer-Chester Medical Center, One Medical Center Blvd, Upland, PA 19013
Phone: (610) 874-6114
Fax: (610) 447-6373
Percentage of IMGs in the program: 0%
Minimum USMLE Step 1 Score Requirement: 213
Minimum USMLE Step 2 Score Requirement: 213
Attempts on any step: No limits set
CS required at time of application: No
USCE Requirement: None
Cut-Off time since graduation: 2 years
Program offers couple match: Yes
Visas Sponsored or accepted: No visa

Reading Health System Transitional Year Residency Program

Specialty: Transitional Year
Program name: Reading Health System Program
Program code: 999-41-00-119
NRMP Code: 1661999P0
Program type: Community-based university affiliated hospital
State: Pennsylvania
Address: Reading Hospital,
       Sixth Ave & Spruce Streets, Reading, PA 19612
Phone: (484) 628-8470
Fax: (484) 628-9003
Percentage of IMGs in the program: 0%
Minimum USMLE Step 1 Score Requirement: 220
Minimum USMLE Step 2 Score Requirement: 220
Attempts on any step: Must pass on first attempt
CS required at time of application: Yes including ECFMG certificate
USCE Requirement: None
Cut-Off time since graduation: No limits set
Program offers couple match: Yes
Visas Sponsored or accepted: J1 visa and H1b visa

South Carolina

Trident Medical Center/Medical University of South Carolina Transitional Year Residency Program

Specialty: Transitional Year
Program name: Trident Medical Center/Medical University of South Carolina Program
Program code: 999-45-00-252
NRMP Code: 2056999P0
Program type: Community-based
State: South Carolina
Address: Trident Med Center,
          9228 Medical Plaza Dr, Charleston, SC 29406
Phone: (843) 876-7080
Fax: (843) 876-7111
Percentage of IMGs in the program: 0%
Minimum USMLE Step 1 Score Requirement: 210
Minimum USMLE Step 2 Score Requirement: 210
Attempts on any step: Must pass on first attempt including CS exam

CS required at time of application: Yes
including ECFMG certificate
USCE Requirement: Yes
Cut-Off time since graduation: 5 years
Program offers couple match: Yes
Visas Sponsored or accepted: J1 visa and H1b
visa

Spartanburg Regional Healthcare System Transitional Year Residency Program

Specialty: Transitional Year
Program name: Spartanburg Regional
Healthcare System Program
Program code: 999-45-00-182
NRMP Code: 1685999P0
Program type: Community-based university
affiliated hospital
State: South Carolina
Address: Spartanburg Regional Healthcare
System,
101 E Wood St, Spartanburg, SC
29303
Phone: (864) 560-6929
Fax: (864) 560-7343
Percentage of IMGs in the program: 0%
Minimum USMLE Step 1 Score Requirement:
No limits set

Minimum USMLE Step 2 Score Requirement:
No limits set
Attempts on any step: No limits set
CS required at time of application: No
USCE Requirement: None
Cut-Off time since graduation: No limits set
Program offers couple match: Yes
Visas Sponsored or accepted: No visa

South Dakota

University of South Dakota Transitional Year Residency Program

Specialty: Transitional Year
Program name: University of South Dakota Program
Program code: 999-46-00-230
NRMP Code: 2805999P0
Program type: Community-based university affiliated hospital
State: South Dakota
Address: USD Sanford School of Medicine,
          1400 W 22nd St, Sioux Falls, SD 57105
Phone: (605) 357-1386
Fax: (605) 357-1548
Percentage of IMGs in the program: 0%

Minimum USMLE Step 1 Score Requirement:
No limits set
Minimum USMLE Step 2 Score Requirement:
No limits set
Attempts on any step: No limits set
CS required at time of application: Yes
including ECFMG certificate
USCE Requirement: None
Cut-Off time since graduation: No limits set
Program offers couple match: Yes
Visas Sponsored or accepted: No visa

Tennessee

University of Tennessee College of Medicine at Chattanooga Transitional Year Residency Program

Specialty: Transitional Year
Program name: University of Tennessee College of Medicine at Chattanooga Program
Program code: 999-47-00-129
NRMP Code: 1689999P0
Program type: University-based
State: Tennessee
Address: University of Tennessee College of Med-Chattanooga,

975 E Third St, Chattanooga, TN 37403
Phone: (423) 778-6670
Fax: (423) 778-2611
Percentage of IMGs in the program: 0%
Minimum USMLE Step 1 Score Requirement: 220
Minimum USMLE Step 2 Score Requirement: 220
Attempts on any step: No limits set
CS required at time of application: Yes including ECFMG certificate
USCE Requirement: None
Cut-Off time since graduation: 5 years
Program offers couple match: Yes
Visas Sponsored or accepted: J1 visa

University of Tennessee Medical Center at Knoxville Transitional Year Residency Program

Specialty: Transitional Year
Program name: University of Tennessee Medical Center at Knoxville Program
Program code: 999-47-00-130
NRMP Code: 1839999P0, 1839999P2
Program type: University-based
State: Tennessee
Address: University of Tennessee Memorial Hospital,

1924 Alcoa Hwy, Knoxville, TN 37920
Phone: (865) 305-9340   Ext: 6501
Fax: (865) 305-6849
Percentage of IMGs in the program: 0%
Minimum USMLE Step 1 Score Requirement:
No limits
Minimum USMLE Step 2 Score Requirement:
No limits
Attempts on any step: Must pass on first
attempt including CS exam
CS required at time of application: Yes
USCE Requirement: Yes
Cut-Off time since graduation: 5 years
Program offers couple match: Yes
Visas Sponsored or accepted: J1 visa

University of Tennessee/Methodist Healthcare-Memphis Hospitals Transitional Year Residency Program

Specialty: Transitional Year
Program name: University of
Tennessee/Methodist Healthcare-Memphis
Hospitals Program
Program code: 999-47-00-131
NRMP Code: 1844999P0
Program type: Community-based university
affiliated hospital
State: Tennessee

Address: Methodist Healthcare-Memphis,
251 S Claybrook, Memphis, TN 38104-3499
Phone: (901) 516-8255
Fax: (901) 516-8254
Percentage of IMGs in the program: 0%
Minimum USMLE Step 1 Score Requirement: No limits set
Minimum USMLE Step 2 Score Requirement: No limits set
Attempts on any step: Must pass on first attempt including CS exam
CS required at time of application: Yes including ECFMG certificate
USCE Requirement: Yes
Cut-Off time since graduation: 2 years
Program offers couple match: Yes
Visas Sponsored or accepted: J1 visa

Texas

University of Texas Southwestern Medical School (Austin) Transitional Year Residency Program

Specialty: Transitional Year

Program name: University of Texas Southwestern Medical School (Austin) Program
Program code: 999-48-00-133
NRMP Code: 2835999P0
Program type: Community-based university affiliated hospital
State: Texas
Address: University of Texas Southwestern Medical School Austin,

      601 E 15th St, Austin, TX 78701
Phone: (512) 324-7997
Fax: (512) 324-7969
Percentage of IMGs in the program: 0%
Minimum USMLE Step 1 Score Requirement: 220
Minimum USMLE Step 2 Score Requirement: 220
Attempts on any step: Must pass on first attempt
CS required at time of application: No
USCE Requirement: None
Cut-Off time since graduation: 5 years
Program offers couple match: Yes
Visas Sponsored or accepted: J1 visa

John Peter Smith Hospital (Tarrant County Hospital District) Transitional Year Residency Program

Specialty: Transitional Year
Program name: John Peter Smith Hospital (Tarrant County Hospital District) Program
Program code: 999-48-00-168
State: Texas
Address: John Peter Smith Hospital, 1500 S Main St, Fort Worth, TX 76104
Phone: (817) 927-1255
Fax: (817) 927-1405
Percentage of IMGs in the program: 0%
Minimum USMLE Step 1 Score Requirement: No limits set
Minimum USMLE Step 2 Score Requirement: No limits set
Attempts on any step: Must pass on first attempt including CS exam
CS required at time of application: Yes
USCE Requirement: None
Cut-Off time since graduation: 2 years
Program offers couple match: Yes
Visas Sponsored or accepted: J1 visa

Methodist Hospital (Houston) Transitional Year Residency Program

Specialty: Transitional Year
Program name: Methodist Hospital (Houston) Program
Program code: 999-48-00-140

NRMP Code: 1167999P0
Program type: Community-based university affiliated hospital
State: Texas
Address: Methodist Hosp Houston,
            6550 Fannin St, Houston, TX 77030
Phone: (713) 441-4431
Fax: (713) 790-6615
Percentage of IMGs in the program: 0%
Minimum USMLE Step 1 Score Requirement: 220
Minimum USMLE Step 2 Score Requirement: 220
Attempts on any step: Must pass on first attempt including CS exam
CS required at time of application: Yes including ECFMG certificate
USCE Requirement: Yes
Cut-Off time since graduation: 2 years unless clinically active as in residency, USCE or practice
Program offers couple match: Yes
Visas Sponsored or accepted: No visa

Utah

Intermountain Medical Center Transitional Year Residency Program

Specialty: Transitional Year
Program name: Intermountain Medical Center Program
Program code: 999-49-00-142
NRMP Code: 1729999P0
Program type: Community-based university affiliated hospital
State: Utah
Address: Intermountain Medical Center, 5169 S Cottonwood St, Murray, UT 84107
Phone: (801) 507-3750
Fax: (801) 507-3799
Percentage of IMGs in the program: 0%
Minimum USMLE Step 1 Score Requirement: 225
Minimum USMLE Step 2 Score Requirement: 225
Attempts on any step: Must pass on first attempt including CS exam
CS required at time of application: Yes including ECFMG Certificate
USCE Requirement: Yes
Cut-Off time since graduation: No limits set
Program offers couple match: Yes
Visas Sponsored or accepted: No visa

Virginia

Georgetown University Hospital Transitional Year Residency Program

Specialty: Transitional Year
Program name: Inova Fairfax Hospital/Georgetown University Program
Program code: 999-51-00-205
State: Virginia
Address: Inova Fairfax Hospital
3300 Gallows Road, Falls Church, VA 22042-3300
Phone: (703) 776-2166
Percentage of IMGs in the program: 0%
Minimum USMLE Step 1 Score Requirement: 210
Minimum USMLE Step 2 Score Requirement: 210
Attempts on any step: No limits set
CS required at time of application: No
USCE Requirement: None
Cut-Off time since graduation: No limits set
Program offers couple match: Yes
Visas Sponsored or accepted: J1 visa

Riverside Regional Medical Center Transitional Year Residency Program

Specialty: Transitional Year
Program name: Riverside Regional Medical Center Program
Program code: 999-51-00-170
NRMP Code: 1739999P0
Program type: Community-based
State: Virginia
Address: Riverside Regional Medical Center, 12200 Warwick Blvd, Newport News, VA 23601-1976
Phone: (757) 534-6112
Fax: (757) 534-6096
Percentage of IMGs in the program: 0%
Minimum USMLE Step 1 Score Requirement: 230
Minimum USMLE Step 2 Score Requirement: 230
Attempts on any step: Must pass on first attempt including the CS exam
CS required at time of application: No
USCE Requirement: None
Cut-Off time since graduation: 2 years unless clinically active as in residency or practice
Program offers couple match: Yes
Visas Sponsored or accepted: J1 visa and H1b visa

Washington

Virginia Mason Medical Center Transitional Year Residency Program

Specialty: Transitional Year
Program name: Virginia Mason Medical Center Program
Program code: 999-54-00-144
NRMP Code: 1756999P0
Program type: Community-based
State: Washington
Address: Virginia Mason Medical Center,
925 Seneca St, Seattle, WA 98101
Phone: (206) 583-6079   Ext: 11296
Percentage of IMGs in the program: 0%
Minimum USMLE Step 1 Score Requirement: No limits set
Minimum USMLE Step 2 Score Requirement: No limits set
Attempts on any step: Must pass on first attempt
CS required at time of application: No
USCE Requirement: No, unless old graduate
Cut-Off time since graduation: 3 years unless clinically active as in residency or practice
Program offers couple match: Yes
Visas Sponsored or accepted: J1 visa

Providence Sacred Heart Medical Center (Spokane) Transitional Year Residency Program

Specialty: Transitional Year
Program name: Providence Sacred Heart Medical Center (Spokane) Program
Program code: 999-54-00-145
NRMP Code: 1758999P0
Program type: Community-based
State: Washington
Address: Providence Sacred Heart Medical Center,
            101 W 8th Ave, Spokane, WA 99204
Phone: (509) 474-3020
Fax: (509) 474-5316
Percentage of IMGs in the program: 0%
Minimum USMLE Step 1 Score Requirement: 225
Minimum USMLE Step 2 Score Requirement: 225
Attempts on any step: Must pass on first attempt
CS required at time of application: No
USCE Requirement: Yes 3 months
Cut-Off time since graduation: 5 years
Program offers couple match: No
Visas Sponsored or accepted: No visa

West Virginia

West Virginia University Transitional Year Residency Program

Specialty: Transitional Year
Program name: West Virginia University Program
Program code: 999-55-00-248
NRMP Code: 1837999P0, 1837999P2
Program type: University-based
State: West Virginia
Address: West Virginia University HSC, One Medical Center Dr, Morgantown, WV 26506
Phone: (304) 293-2463
Percentage of IMGs in the program: 0%
Minimum USMLE Step 1 Score Requirement: 210
Minimum USMLE Step 2 Score Requirement: 210
Attempts on any step: Must pass on first attempt including CS exam
CS required at time of application: Yes including ECFMG certificate
USCE Requirement: None
Cut-Off time since graduation: No limits set
Program offers couple match: Yes
Visas Sponsored or accepted: J1 visa

Wisconsin

Gundersen Lutheran Medical Foundation Transitional Year Residency Program

Specialty: Transitional Year
Program name: Gundersen Lutheran Medical Foundation Program
Program code: 999-56-00-147
State: Wisconsin
Address: Gundersen Medical Foundation, 1836 South Ave, La Crosse, WI 54601-5429
Phone: (608) 775-2961 Ext: 52961
Fax: (608) 775-1548
Percentage of IMGs in the program: 0%
Minimum USMLE Step 1 Score Requirement: No limits set
Minimum USMLE Step 2 Score Requirement: No limits set
Attempts on any step: Must pass on first attempt including CS exam
CS required at time of application: Yes including ECFMG certificate
USCE Requirement: None
Cut-Off time since graduation: 2 years

Program offers couple match: Yes
Visas Sponsored or accepted: J1 visa and H1b visa

Marshfield Clinic-St Joseph Hospital Transitional Year Residency Program

Specialty: Transitional Year
Program name: Marshfield Clinic-St Joseph's Hospital Program
Program code: 999-56-00-183
NRMP Code: 1780999P0
Program type: Community-based university affiliated hospital
State: Wisconsin
Address: Marshfield Clinic,
            1000 N Oak Ave, Marshfield, WI 54449
Phone: (715) 389-4151
Fax: (715) 389-4141
Percentage of IMGs in the program: 20%
Minimum USMLE Step 1 Score Requirement: 210
Minimum USMLE Step 2 Score Requirement: 210
Attempts on any step: No limits set
CS required at time of application: No
USCE Requirement: Yes
Cut-Off time since graduation: 3 years

Program offers couple match: Yes
Visas Sponsored or accepted: J1 visa and H1b visa

Aurora Health Care Transitional Year Residency Program

Specialty: Transitional Year
Program name: Aurora Health Care Program
Program code: 999-56-00-148
NRMP Code: 1789999P0
Program type: Community-based university affiliated hospital
State: Wisconsin
Address: Aurora St Luke's Hospital,
          2801 W Kinnickinnic River Pkwy,
Milwaukee, WI 53215
Phone: (414) 649-3323
Fax: (414) 649-5158
Percentage of IMGs in the program: 0%
Minimum USMLE Step 1 Score Requirement: 205
Minimum USMLE Step 2 Score Requirement: 205
Attempts on any step: Maximum of 3 attempts on each step including CS exam
CS required at time of application: No
USCE Requirement: None unless old graduate
Cut-Off time since graduation: 5 years unless clinically active as in residency or practice

Program offers couple match: Yes
Visas Sponsored or accepted: J1 visa

Wheaton Franciscan Healthcare-St Joseph Transitional Year Residency Program

Specialty: Transitional Year
Program name: Wheaton Franciscan Healthcare-St Joseph Program
Program code: 999-56-00-184
NRMP Code: 1788999P0
Program type: Community-based university affiliated hospital
State: Wisconsin
Address: Wheaton Franciscan-St Joseph,
        5000 W Chambers St, Milwaukee, WI 53210
Phone: (414) 447-2195
Fax: (414) 874-4533
Percentage of IMGs in the program: 0%
Minimum USMLE Step 1 Score Requirement: 215
Minimum USMLE Step 2 Score Requirement: No limits set
Attempts on any step: No limits set
CS required at time of application: No
USCE Requirement: None but must be clinically active if graduated a long time
Cut-Off time since graduation: No limits set

Program offers couple match: Yes
Visas Sponsored or accepted: No visa

I wish you good luck.

Thank you for buying our book.

Please, Please and Please take a minute to review our book on Amazon.

Match A Doc
Residency Guide